Diabetes Military Coup:

Guaranteed Method of Controlling Your Glucose Levels

By

Dr. Elizabeth M. Harris

TABLE OF CONTENTS

INTRODUCTION

A sugar levels test analyzes the sugar levels in your blood. Glucose is a kind of sugar. It is your body's principal source of energy. A hormone known as insulin helps transfer glucose from your circulation into your cells. In excess or insufficient glucose in the body might be a symptom of a dangerous medical issue. Having high blood sugar levels could be the indication of diabetic, a sickness which may cause considerable, protracted health concerns. High blood sugar may also be caused by other disorders that might impact insulin or sugar levels in your blood, such as issues with your pancreas or adrenal glands.

Lower blood sugar levels (hypoglycemia) are prevalent between persons with type 1 diabetes and those with type 2 diabetes who use specific diabetic drugs. Certain illnesses, such as liver disease, may generate low levels of blood sugar levels in persons without diabetes, although this is unusual. Without treatment, extreme low blood sugar may lead to grave health concerns, such seizures and head trauma.

Chapter 1

What is Glucose?

While your glucose levels are effectively maintained, they typically go undetected. However, they might disrupt your body's everyday functioning when they fall too low or become too high.

What is, therefore, Glucose, precisely?

It's the essential carbohydrate (carb), making it a simple sugars, implying "one sugar." Additional simple sugar include fructose, lactose, and ribose. In this state, ingested Glucose or other carbs ultimately transform into blood sugar in the body. Alongside protein and fat, Glucose is one of the body's principal fuel sources. People may obtain Glucose from complicated and simple carb origins.Carbs are simple and complicated depending on how rapidly the system aids the digestion of the Glucose. Analysis shows the body digests complex carbs more slowly, giving them a more constant renewable resource. This makes them a healthier decision. Unmanaged glucose levels may have lifelong and catastrophic repercussions.

How does the body process glucose?

Your body optimally utilizes Glucose many times a day. When you eat, it rapidly begins functioning to digest Glucose and other carbs. Then, enzymes start to break them down with support from the pancreas. The pancreas, which generates hormones like insulin, is vital to how your body deals with Glucose, according to a 2021 study by Trusted Source. When you eat, your body urges the pancreas to produce insulin to regulate the growing blood sugar level. Muscle, fat, and other cells then utilize Glucose for energy or store it as fat for later use. Diabetes could arise when the pancreas doesn't generate insulin the way it should. In this instance, you may require outside intervention (insulin injections) to digest and control Glucose in the body. A 2018 analysis reveals that diabetes may potentially result from insulin resistance. This occurs when the body's cells do not perceive insulin, and too much sugar stays in circulation. When the body does not react to insulin the way it should, it inhibits Glucose from entering your cells and being utilized for energy. Your cells respond by signaling the synthesis of ketones at night and during fasting or dieting.

How can diabetes tests discriminate between Glucose and other sugars in the blood?

Blood sugar, or Glucose, is the significant sugar in your blood. Your blood transports Glucose to all of your body's cells to consume energy. Diabetes is a disease in which your glucose levels are excessively high. Over time, having too much Glucose in your blood might create significant complications. Three blood tests are the most reliable for identifying prediabetes and diabetes: The fasting plasma glucose test checks blood sugar levels after an overnight fast (eight to 12 hours) and has been the standard first diagnostic approach for decades. Go to my profile, and you may discover all Diabetes content there...

Over time, with insulin resistance, your insulin levels may become low, according to the American Diabetes Association (ADA). Your body may also release fat from fat cells. In addition, the liver continues generating additional ketones, decreasing your blood pH to an acidic level. The ADA says that when your body cannot utilize Glucose as it needs to, the development of ketones and shift in blood pH may become harmful. This occurrence is known as ketoacidosis. It is a severe and life-or-death consequence of diabetes which thus demands prompt medical treatment.

How do our systems "vaporize" Glucose to generate energy?

Our body requires Glucose to gain the necessary energy to function. Glucose is acquired mainly by the body via ingesting carbs. Each gram of carbs you eat contains four calories containing energy. After being absorbed by the body, specific enzymes in the digestive tract break down the carbs you have consumed into simple sugars called Glucose. This down tearing process enables the body to obtain the calories of energy included inside the carbohydrates.

Insulin

After consuming a meal, the body begins to work to decompose the carbs to make Glucose. The blood sugar levels are released into the bloodstream and boost your blood sugar levels. For the cells to acquire Glucose in circulation, your pancreas must generate a hormone known as insulin. As your blood glucose levels rise, the pancreas is prompted to produce insulin into circulation. Absent insulin, your cells will struggle to absorb the Glucose needed for energy. Problems with insulin can develop due to a lack of insulin created by the system, or the organisms have grown resistant to it. These difficulties are signs of an illness called diabetes. When insufficient insulin is produced, this may result in a dramatically low blood glucose level, which renders the cells unable to make enough power to live. If the partitions develop insulin resistance, this may lead to too much Glucose in the circulation, which can cause catastrophic damage to the body's blood vessels.

Receptors

Every cell in your body has unique machinery in them called insulin receptors. These receptors can attach to insulin when they come into contact. This binding functions as a key to unlocking the cell's capacity to take Glucose out of circulation and into the cell itself. This is done via the glucose transporter molecules in the cell's membrane.

Cell Metabolism

Once Glucose has penetrated the cell, the cell attempts to tear the Glucose to generate energy. This is accomplished by a mechanism called aerobic metabolism. During aerobic metabolism, oxygen is taken out of the blood and delivered to the cell with Glucose. The mitochondria utilize oxygen to convert Glucose into thermal energy and adenosine triphosphate (ATP) (ATP). ATP is subsequently used to store or let the energy generated based on the cell's demands.

Chapter 2
Glucose Testing

The Role of Glucose Testing

There are different reasons a doctor could prescribe glucose testing for you, including screening, diagnosis, and observing.

Screening

Screening implies testing to detect health concerns before those problems develop any symptoms or indicators you or your doctor could notice. If you're over 40, overweight or obese, or have an elevated risk of developing diabetes, your doctor may recommend one or more screening glucose tests to discover prediabetes or diabetes.

Diagnosis

Diagnosis involves experiments and procedures to discover what underlying health issue could generate obvious indications and symptoms.

If you experience symptoms of diabetes, high blood sugar, or low blood sugar, your doctor may recommend glucose testing for you. Glucose testing may be supplemented by additional blood or urine tests to provide an accurate analysis.

Observing

Assuming you have been diagnosed with diabetes or prediabetes, your doctor may want you to follow your blood glucose levels using at-home glucose testing or monitoring equipment. Your doctor may also suggest frequent laboratory tests at checkups to understand how your disease is being controlled.

Who should receive the test?

Your doctor may also want to check you for increased glucose tolerance if you have a higher-than-average risk of diabetes. Risk factors for diabetes include \s• Being 45 years of age or older \s• Being overweight or obese \s• Heart disease, high blood pressure, or high cholesterol s• Prediabetes \s• Having family members with diabetes s• A lack of physical activity \s• African American, Asian, Hispanic, or Native American/American Indian ethnicity s• Polycystic ovarian syndrome.

Assuming you is pregnant, your doctor may recommend glucose tests to check for gestational diabetes, a form of diabetes related to hormone changes during pregnancy. Having gestational diabetes may be hazardous to the mother and baby if left untreated and can raise your risk of diabetes later in life.

Feeling your doctor may also recommend glucose testing if you are experiencing symptoms of diabetes, including s• Frequent urination \s•

Excessive hunger or thirst \s• Tingling or loss of Feeling in the hands or feet \, s• Blurred vision \s• an odd number of infections \s• Unexplained weight loss \s• Feeling fatigued \s• Skin that is dry \s• Sores that don't heal quickly \s• feeling very tired.

Additionally, your doctor may recommend glucose testing if you have symptoms of low blood sugar or other health concerns. Glucose testing is also an essential aspect of controlling prediabetes and diabetes when they are identified.

Types of Glucose Tests

Numerous different glucose tests are regularly used for evaluating and diagnosing.

• **Fasting blood glucose test**: This test measures the quantity of Glucose in the bloodstream after you've gone without eating or drinking anything except water for at least 12 hours. This test is usually administered in the morning.

• **Random plasma glucose test**: This test likewise evaluates the quantity of Glucose in the blood but may be conducted at any time of the day, whether or not you've eaten lately. It is frequently done on a sample of blood obtained from a vein in your arm and may be included in a panel of blood tests, such as a complete absorption panel. People treated with diabetes may also test their Glucose throughout the day using a finger stick blood sample and specific equipment that offers results at home.

• **Glucose tolerance test**: This test examines how much Glucose is in your system after you fast overnight and then consume a sweet drink. A glucose tolerance test often requires more than one blood collection over several hours.

• **Urine glucose test**: Urine glucose testing is commonly part of regular urinalysis. A urine analysis tests for the presence of numerous chemicals in the urine. Urine glucose test findings are less reliable than blood glucose testing. Your specialist might recommend this test if you cannot undergo a blood test.

• **Continuous glucose monitoring**: A continuous glucose monitor monitors glucose levels using a small wire inserted just below the skin's surface. This form of monitoring may indicate blood glucose trends over time.

• **Hemoglobin A1C**: Whereas the hemoglobin A1C test does not directly detect Glucose, it does indicate your typical blood glucose levels over the last three months by assessing the amount of hemoglobin attached Glucose.

Although glucose tests most typically employ blood or urine samples to screen for and monitor diabetes, they may also be conducted on samples of cerebrospinal fluid (CSF) or joint fluid. Abnormal amounts of Glucose in the CSF or synovial membrane may be due to the virus, bacterial or fungal infections, and other diseases.

If you receive abnormal findings on a glucose test, your doctor may want to repeat the test or have you take a different kind of glucose test to validate the results. Depending on your case, the sort of glucose test your doctor may prescribe, how frequently it's administered, when and where you will have the test, and if you need extra testing.

Getting Glucose Testing

Glucose testing for screening and diagnosis occurs at a doctor's office, clinic, or laboratory. Plasma glucose testing entails collecting blood from a vein using a tiny needle. Urinalysis includes collecting a fresh sample of urine in a specimen cup. Your doctor may explain which tests are the most suited for your circumstances, let you know if you will need to fast before the test and how much time it will take, and offer you further advice about preparing for it.

At-home testing

Screening and diagnostic glucose testing are not done at home. But if you've been treated for diabetes, you may have to stay on top of your blood glucose level using at-home tests. At-home monitoring helps you and your doctor understand how effectively your diabetes is being managed and may help you make treatment options if your glucose levels are too high or too low. At-home blood glucose testing has been most typically done with a glucose meter. Furthermore, your doctor may suggest you utilize continuous glucose monitoring to assess your blood sugar at home. If you check your glucose levels at home, you may still need to check your blood glucose occasionally in a clinical environment. Your doctor may tell you which at-home tests or tests are suitable for you and may be able to recommend particular brands or test kits.

Chapter 3

What triggers low blood sugar?

Low blood sugar (also termed hypoglycemia) has several causes, including skipping a meal, excessive use of insulin, taking additional diabetic treatments, exercising more than usual, and consuming alcohol. If your Glucose is below 70 mg/dB is considered as low.

Symptoms of low blood sugar levels are varied for everyone. Main signs include:

• Shaking.

• Sweating.

• Nervousness or anxiety.

• Irritability or confusion.

• Dizziness.

• Hunger.

Know your specific symptoms so you can recognize low blood sugar early and cure it. If you believe you may have low blood sugar, check it even if you don't have symptoms. Low blood sugar may be harmful and should be addressed quickly.

How, then, can I cure low blood sugar?

Carry things for treating low blood sugar with you. Check your blood sugar if you feel shaky, hot, starving, or have other symptoms. Even if you don't have symptoms but suspect you may have low blood sugar, examine it. If your blood sugar is fewer than 70 mg/dB, perform one of the following immediately:

• Take four glucose pills.

• Drink four ounces of fruit juice.

• Drink four ounces of ordinary soda, not diet soda.

• Eat four pieces of hard candy.

Stop for 15 minutes, and then recheck your blood sugar. Perform one of the above medications until your blood sugar is 70 mg/dB or above, and have a snack when your next meal is an hour away. Whether you encounter difficulties with low blood sugar, inquire with your doctor if your treatment regimen needs to be adjusted.

What drives blood glucose to be high?

Many reasons may induce high blood sugar (hyperglycemia), such as being unwell, anxious, eating more than expected, and not giving oneself enough insulin. Over time, elevated blood sugar may lead to long-term, significant health concerns. Symptoms of high blood sugar include:

• Feeling exhausted.

• Feeling thirsty.

• Having hazy eyesight.

• Needing to urinate (pee) excessively frequently.

If you are ill, your blood sugar might be challenging to regulate. You may not be able to eat or drink as much as standard, which might influence blood sugar levels. If you're unwell and your blood sugar is 240 mg/dB or higher, use an over-the-counter ketone test kit to check your urine for ketones and contact your doctor if your ketones are elevated. High ketones may be an early symptom of diabetic ketoacidosis, a medical emergency that must be treated quickly.

What are ketones?

Ketones are a fuel created when fat is broken down for energy. Your liver begins breaking down fat when there's insufficient insulin in your circulation to get blood sugar to enter your cells.

Diabetic ketoacidosis

When too many ketones are created too rapidly, they may pile up in your body and cause diabetic ketoacidosis, or DKA. DKA is quite dangerous and may induce a coma or even death. Typical symptoms of DKA include:

• Fast, deep breathing.

• Skin problems and breathe.

• Flushed face.

• Regular peeing or thirst that should last for a day or longer.

• Fruity-smelling breath.

• Headache.

• Muscle tightness or aches.

• Nausea and vomiting.

• Stomach discomfort.

If you believe you may have DKA, test your urine for ketones. Follow the test kit guidelines, verifying the color of the test strip against the color chart in the kit to find your ketone level. If your ketones are high, contact your health care practitioner straight away. DKA needs treatment in a hospital.DKA happens primarily in patients with type 1 diabetes and is frequently the first indicator of type 1 in those who haven't yet been diagnosed. People with type 2 diabetes may also get DKA, although it's less frequent.

How can I cure high blood sugar?

Talk to your doctor about ways to maintain your blood sugar levels within your goal range. Your doctor may advise the following:

• Be more active. Regular exercise might help keep your blood sugar levels in balance. Important: don't exercise if ketones are detected in your urine. This might make your blood sugar go even higher.

• Take the medicine as instructed. If your blood sugar is regularly high, your doctor may adjust how much medication you take or when you take it.

• Follow your diabetic food plan. Ask your doctor or dietician for advice if you're having problems adhering to it.

• Check your blood sugar as advised by your doctor. Check regularly if you're unwell or worried about high or low blood sugar.

• Talk to your doctor about modifying how much insulin you take and what kinds of insulin (such as short-acting) to use.

How do carbohydrates impact blood sugar?

Carbs in meals cause your blood sugar levels to increase more after consuming them than when you eat proteins or fats. You can still consume carbohydrates if you have diabetes. The quantity you can drink and remain in your target blood sugar range depends on your age, weight, exercise level, and other variables. Counting carbohydrates in meals and beverages is essential for regulating blood sugar levels. Make sure to chat to your health care provider about your optimal carb targets.

What is the A1C test?

The A1C test is a basic blood test that evaluates your average blood sugar levels over the preceding 2 or 3 months. The test is done in a lab or your doctor's office in addition to not instead of regular blood sugar testing you perform yourself. A1C testing is one of the ABCs of diabetes essential actions you may take to avoid or delay health concerns on the road:

• A: Get a regular A1C test.

• B: Try to maintain your blood pressure below 140/90 mm Hg (or the goal your doctor sets) (or the target your doctor sets).

• C: Manage your cholesterol levels.

• S: Stop smoking or don't start.

The A1C target for most individuals with diabetes is between 7% and 8%, although your goal may differ based on your age, underlying health problems, drugs, and other variables. Work with your doctor to develop a customized A1C target for you.

What else can I do to regulate my blood sugar levels?

Taking a balanced diet with lots of fruit and vegetables, keeping a healthy weight, and regular physical exercise may help. Other tips include:

• Keep track of your blood sugar levels to observe what causes them to increase or decrease.

• Eat at regular times, and don't miss meals.

• Choose foods lower in calories, saturated fat, Trans fat, sugar, and salt.

• Track your food, drink, and physical activity.

• Drink water instead of juice or soda.

• Limit alcoholic beverages.

• For a sweet treat, select fruit.

• Restrict your meal amounts (for instance, utilize the titration method: fill half your plate with non-starchy veggies, a fourth with high-quality protein, and a part with a grain or starchy items)

Chapter 4

How or when to Normalize Your Blood Sugar?

Maintaining control of blood sugar levels is crucial for treating type 2 diabetes. Here's how to handle this often tricky course of diabetes treatment. Life with type 2 diabetes may often feel like an hourly or minute-by-minute battle to control your blood sugar. All of the suggestions and medicines you've been given as components of your type 2 diabetes treatment plan are meant to help you attain and stay healthy blood sugar levels most of the time. But physicians realize that to handle type 2 diabetes successfully, a greater understanding of why blood sugar matters and how to manage it is vital.

Shocking Realities regarding Diabetes and Blood Glucose

As the American Diabetes Association (ADA) describes, your body requires sugar (Glucose) for energy, and a rather sophisticated procedure makes it feasible for your body to utilize that sugar. Insulin, created by the pancreas, is the hormone that allows the organs and tissues to take advantage of sugar. Type 2 diabetes occurs when your body isn't capable of removing sugar from your blood. This may happen if your body ceases being responsive to insulin or begins to react in a delayed or excessive manner to fluctuations in your blood sugar. Diabetes is signified by an increased blood sugar level exceeding 126 milligrams per deciliter (mg/dB) for an overnight blood test or more than 200 mg/dB at any point throughout the day. It may also be suggested by a hemoglobin A1C level of 6.5 per cent or above, measuring the amount of blood sugar bound to hemoglobin in the blood over the last two to three months. (Hemoglobin is a protein in red blood cells that distributes oxygen throughout the body. So an A1C of 6.5 signifies that 6.5 per cent of your red blood cells have sugar linked to them.)Uncontrolled high blood sugar eventually destroys the capillaries in your body. Over the long run, this gradual, increasing injury may lead to a severe loss of feeling in your legs and feet, a loss of vision and renal function, and an elevated risk for heart disease and stroke. Two very different high and low blood sugar are medical challenges. "Low blood sugar may result in hypoglycemia, which puts individuals at risk for disorientation and loss of consciousness. Therefore it can be life-threatening.

Techniques to help strengthen Glucose Levels.

Increasing your glucose levels to sustainable levels may involve experimentation, but there are measures to help you do it.

"A daily routine is crucial for excellent diabetes management that entails following your diet plan, exercising consistently, being persistent with blood glucose monitoring, and following up often with your doctor." Tracking carbs is very crucial. "Big differences in carbohydrate consumption from day to day might contribute to oscillations in blood sugars," she says. For example, when you take extra carbs, the body digests them like sugar and transfers them directly into the circulation, increasing the risk of blood sugar.

Follow these precise measures to help regulate blood sugar:

Exercise: A regular exercise regimen has been demonstrated to help regulate blood sugar levels over time. A diversified fitness approach is helpful for diabetes and health in general. Participants in a 12-week program who exercised for an hour three times a week utilizing both aerobic and resistance training had better diabetes control, according to a study published in February 2015 in the Journal of Sports Medicine and Physical Fitness. So mix it up with weight training, cardio exercises, and other things you love. Weight Loss If you're overweight, it will be simpler to balance blood sugar more successfully if you shed even a few pounds. "For most persons with diabetes, decreasing only 5 or 10 pounds may make a difference in diabetes management or the requirement for medication. Diet, many persons with diabetes acquire greater control over their blood sugar by reducing the sorts of meals that might cause blood sugar to increase. For example, your doctor could suggest cutting down on carbs and eating more lean protein, fruits, and vegetables. Fiber may be so valuable that putting even a fair bit of a fiber supplement into a meal that ordinarily could elevate blood sugar will help stabilize it. Drinking Wisely Alcohol may induce an instant spike in blood sugar and a reduction a few hours later. It's advisable to keep to modest portions and have some substantial food with your drinks Medication, your doctor may offer various kinds of medicine at different Stages throughout your diabetes therapy. Treatment options include the following:

• Iguanids', the medicine family that includes metformin, help your body utilize insulin more efficiently and may also lower the amount of blood sugar generated by the liver.

• Sulfonylureas stimulate some cells in your pancreas to create more insulin, while low blood sugar (hypoglycemia) is a potential adverse effect.

• Meglitinides, a family of medications that includes repaginate, stimulate your pancreas to create more insulin, with hypoglycemia as a potential adverse effect.

• Thiazolidinedione's, a family that includes approximately 1–2, may help insulin operate effectively.

• Alpha-glycosidase inhibitors, a class containing acerbate, hinder the body from breaking down carbohydrates and may be used to avoid a surge in blood sugar after a meal.

• DPP-4 inhibitors enable GLP-1, a gut-based hormone naturally occurring in the body, to linger longer and help regulate blood sugar levels.

• SGLT2 inhibitors cause extra Glucose to be excreted in the urine.

• Insulin may be essential to help your body utilize blood sugar more efficiently.

How Self - adjusting Blood Glucose Plays a Big Role in Weight Reduction

Our blood sugar level is the assessment of glucose concentration in the blood. The body absorbs Glucose from the food we consume and is the primary energy source in the body. The absorption, storage, and synthesis of Glucose are controlled continually by complicated mechanisms involving the small intestine, liver, and pancreas. The pancreas creates insulin, releasing it when a person eats protein or carbs. The insulin transmits excess Glucose in the liver as glycogen. The pancreas also generates a hormone called glucagon, which performs the opposite of insulin, boosting blood sugar levels when required. When the body needs additional sugar in circulation, the glucagon tells the liver to transform the glycogen back into Glucose and release it into the bloodstream. Whenever your nutrition is in harmony, various systems operate in unison. The issue happens when the body lacks insulin, is consuming too much, or when the body is not working appropriately. Cells may acquire resistance to insulin, resulting in the need for the pancreas to generate and produce more insulin to reduce your blood glucose levels.

Ultimately, the system might fail to have sufficient insulin to catch pace with the Glucose pouring into the system.

How, then, can elevated blood sugar inhibit weight loss?

Weight loss occurs when we spend more energy than we ingest (calories) (calories). But it also happens when we have balanced blood sugar and no extra insulin. Excess insulin is formed as a consequence of too much sugar in our systems. This insulin spike informs our systems that sufficient energy is accessible and that they should stop burning calories and start storing them. By managing your levels and maintaining them in the healthy range (between 80 mg/ml and 120 mg/ml), you will use carbs and proteins for energy rather than storing them as fat.

Foods that help regulate your glucose levels.

The most straightforward strategy to regulate your blood sugar levels is to be conscious of what you consume. Sugar lurks in a lot of our food, particularly if it is prepared. When you concentrate on eating whole foods (items that are mainly produced from the ground), you will have a much better blood sugar level. Eating on a regular schedule and not missing meals is also crucial, so you don't experience a blood sugar drop and look for a processed snack to lift you back up.

WHOLE FRUITS

Specifically, ingesting blueberry, grapes, and apples may help dramatically lessen your chances of getting Type 2 diabetes, 2013 research indicates. In addition to watermelon and plantains, most fruits have low glycemic index (GI) ratings and are an excellent option for regulating glucose levels.

SWEET POTATOES AND YAMS

Sweet potatoes may assist in balancing or reducing blood sugar levels, and they are indeed a good, nutritious meal with a low GI score. People may replace sweet potatoes or yams for potatoes in various meals, from fries to casseroles.

WHOLE WHEAT OR PUMPERNICKEL BREAD

That's right, bread. Even if most loaves should be ignored while balancing blood sugar because of the carbs, entire wheat and pumpernickel possess lower GI scores because they go towards less manufacturing, leaving them with more fiber that slows digestion and contributes to balancing glucose levels.

OATS

Oats are a fantastic food. They lower high insulin response after meals, enhance insulin sensitivity, maintain glycemic control, and reduce lipids in the blood.

NUTS \ Most nuts make a healthful and low GI snack great for making you feel full, giving you energy, and without increasing blood sugar. Nuts also include large quantities of plant proteins, unsaturated fatty acids, and other nutrients, including antioxidants and potassium.

LEGUMES

Beans, chickpeas, peas, and lentils are all legumes that provide fiber, protein, and complex carbs to give you energy, help you feel full longer, and even lessen the risk of coronary heart disease. Be cautious about consuming your beans whole. For example, prepare a pot of beans at home instead. You are opening a can. Those canned and prepared beans might contain heaps of hidden sugar that will undoubtedly disrupt your blood sugar levels.

GARLIC

Garlic has been a medicinal element for hundreds of years in human history, and it is a spicy weapon in the battle against unhealthy blood sugar levels. You may eat it raw, add it to your favorite cuisine, or use it in a homemade dressing; the choices are unlimited!

YOGURT

Ordinary milk or Greek yoghurt has a low GI score and is a decent option for less healthful choices like sour cream or crème fresh. If you can't handle unsweetened yoghurt, consider adding a natural sweetener like honey or a low GI fruit like blueberries.

Understanding your body's method of storing sugar and listening to your body's demands can assist in general health and optimum performance. While your total calorie intake is vital when you are seeking to lose weight, monitoring your sugar consumption will offer you extraordinary results sooner. And you will be constructing a healthier physique overall.

Advantages of Balanced Blood Glucose: How else to Obtain and Maintain each one.

Have you ever suffered a sugar crash?

Maybe you eat a huge dessert or drink a coke with lunch. Your blood glucose surges, and you feel great for about half an hour, with lots of energy, a good attitude, and so on. But soon, the sugar high goes off. Brain fog makes it hard to concentrate. Your energy takes a dip. You're angry and cranky. Maybe you're plagued with food cravings even if you just ate. If you've ever crashed after consuming sugar or processed carbohydrates, you know what it's like to have to fluctuate blood sugar levels.

Your blood glucose affects you're: Brain function, mental focus, Energy level Mood Hunger and food cravings risk of disease. When you're in excellent condition, your body can cope with the rare surge in blood glucose. But if your blood sugar is on a continual rollercoaster of highs and lows due to your food, age, heredity, and other factors, it may leave you weary, cranky, and hungry throughout the day.

The encouraging news: you can regulate your sugar levels with a few easy lifestyle modifications.

Four Advantages of Steady Glucose

You frequently hear about blood glucose in the situation of diabetes.

But even if you don't have diabetes, balancing your blood sugar is a great way to live longer, enhance your attitude and energy levels, and lose weight more quickly.

Here are four main advantages that come from maintaining your glucose levels constant.

Stable Energy

Processed carbs break down relatively readily in your body. They're already so close to Glucose that you scarcely need to digest them.

Processed carbs speed through digestion and get directly to your bloodstream. Sugar-rich blood travels around your body, and your cells may hold as much of it as they need.

However, elevated blood sugar might be an issue if it lasts too long. Your body recognizes that, so it produces insulin when it detects loads of Glucose in your circulation. This hormone guides sugar out of your blood and into your cells and puts your blood glucose back within an average limit.

This approach works nicely for modest blood sugar rises. You consume some slow-digesting carbohydrates, your blood sugar rises, you produce a little insulin, and your blood sugar lowers back to normal.

But your insulin response may be incorrect if you feel tired after a carb-rich meal. Many individuals don't handle carbohydrates well and have difficulties releasing the proper quantity of insulin at the right time; instead, they put out more insulin than they need and remove it late.

The outcome is low blood sugar, which may leave you exhausted and unable to remain focused.

This yo-yo effect explains how blood sugar changes mess with your energy levels. You swing from an energy-rich high to an energy-poor low instead of sticking in the center and having constant, continuous energy throughout the day.

• In a 2017 study, researchers placed participants on high-glycemic and low-glycemic diets for 28 days. People on high-glycemic diets that generate changes in blood sugar exhibited considerably higher depressive symptoms, mood swings, and fatigue.

People on high-glycemic diets that generate changes in blood sugar exhibited considerably higher depressive symptoms, mood swings, and fatigue. A 2019 study review showed similar results: participants suffered sleepiness and reduced alertness within an hour after consuming refined carbohydrates.

If you are drowsy and have difficulties concentrating after meals, try cutting down on Glucose and other sugary foods. Doing so will regulate your blood glucose and increase your energy.

Sustainable Weight Loss

A healthy brain contains special cells that sense your blood sugar level and change your desires accordingly. If your blood glucose is low, your brain sends signals to induce you to eat more, but if your blood sugar remains consistent, your brain tells your body that you're full, lessening your hunger levels.

In other words, changes in blood sugar might make you feel hungry, making you more inclined to overeat.

On top of that, high-glycemic meals, which upset your blood sugar levels most, are incredibly satisfying and may provoke significant food cravings.

In a 2013 study, males ate either a minimal or elevated dinner. The guys who ate the formal dinner had low blood sugar after that and reported much-increased food cravings.

There was another surprising finding: brain scans indicated that when the guys ate high-glycemic meals, the reward areas of their brains lit up approximately an hour after dinner, just when the participants' cravings started.

Foods that raise your blood glucose are typically tremendously satisfying. They stimulate the pleasure centers of your brain, which is great during the meal, but when that part of your brain loses power, you're left wanting more. That's because more and more evidence shows that high-glycemic meals contribute to food addiction and obesity.

On the other hand, nutrients that keep blood sugar stable, like reduced or low-carb diets, actually decrease food cravings. Not surprisingly, medications also work better for protracted weight loss.

If you're attempting to lose weight, but emotional eating keeps undermining you, consider balancing your blood sugar to attain your fitness objectives.

Mental Clarity

Blood sugar impacts your brain, too. Unstable blood sugar lowers alertness4 and causes emotional swings and mood disorders.

Spikes in blood sugar are also connected to subtle brain injuries. A 2015 research indicated that poor blood sugar regulation relates to lower concentration, lapses in memory, and depletion of grey matter (a significant component of the brain), even in young people without diabetes.

More long-term, frequently high blood sugar may lead to dementia, notably Alzheimer's. Some experts term Alzheimer's "type 3 diabetes" because of the association between fluctuating blood sugar and brain degeneration. For perspective, roughly 35% of Americans have poor blood sugar control without diabetes, and about 84% of people with poor blood sugar control don't recognize that they have it.

By balancing your blood sugar, you can keep your brain healthy, both in the short-term and long-term.

Longevity

Stable blood sugar may fight off dementia and keep your brain healthy far into old age. But it's not the only way that blood sugar influences lifespan.

If you frequently elevate your blood glucose over time, you might begin to develop insulin resistance. Your body, confused by the continual up-and-down in your blood sugar, starts misjudging how much insulin you need to keep your blood sugar steady.

Sometimes it releases too much insulin, other times, it removes too little, and as time goes on, you lose your ability to stabilize your blood sugar. Stable blood sugar maintains your body's receptivity to insulin and minimizes your risk of illness, particularly as you age.

Things that trigger blood sugar

10 Shocking Things That Can Spike Your Blood Sugar

When you initially discovered diabetes, you checked your blood sugar regularly. Doing so helps you understand how food, exercise, stress, and sickness may impact your blood sugar levels. For the most part, you've got it figured out by now. But then bam! Something causes your blood sugar to fly up.

Knowledge is power! Look out for these surprising causes that might send your blood sugar soaring:

1. Sunburn—the discomfort produces stress, and stress raises blood sugar levels.

2. Artificial sweeteners: more study is required, although some studies suggest they may boost blood sugar.

3. Coffee—even without sweetness. Some people's Glucose is extra-sensitive to caffeine.

4. Not sleeping—even just one night of too little sleep might make your body manage insulin less effectively.

5. Skipping breakfast—going without that morning meal might boost blood sugar after lunch and supper.

6. Time of day—blood sugar might be tougher to manage the later it gets.

7. People experience a rise in hormones early in the morning, whether they have diabetes or not. For patients with diabetes, blood sugar might increase.

8. Dehydration—less water in your body means your blood sugar is more concentrated.

9. Nose spray—some include ingredients that encourage your liver to generate more blood sugar.

10. Gum disease—it's both a consequence of diabetes and a blood sugar spike.

Conclusion

Blood glucose concentration, or sugar, is the primary carbohydrate in your bloodstream. It emanates first from the meals you ingest. It is your body's principal energy source. Your blood carries glucose to your body's cells to consume for energy. Diabetes is a condition in which your glucose levels are abnormally high. Over time, having too much sugar in your blood could lead to major difficulties. Even if you don't have diabetes, periodically, you may have concerns with blood glucose levels that are too low or high. Maintaining a regimen of eating, exercising, and taking any essential medications will benefit.

Assuming you have diabetes, it is vital to maintain your blood sugar values in your goal range. You might need to monitor your glucose many times each day. Your healthcare system doctor will also do a blood physical exam and an A1C. It examines your typical blood sugar levels over the last 4 months. If your metabolism is very high, you may need to take medicine and stick to a specific diet.